Low Fodmap Diet

Complete Plans And Simple Recipes For Real Weight Loss
And A Healthy Digestive System

*(Meal Plans And Low-Fodmap Recipes For Relieving And
Healing IBS)*

Clarence Thompson

TABLE OF CONTENT

Chapter 1: What Is The Fodmap-Restricted Diet?

The Low FODMAP diet, despite its name, is not a weight loss regimen. The diet is best undertaken with the assistance of a dietitian or healthcare professional, and begins with a two-to-six-week period of strict calorie restriction. Then, certain foods can typically be reintroduced.

In hort, FODMAP are a group of roorlu-aborbed fermentable short-chain carbohydrates that can result in excessive fluid and gas production, frequently causing gastrointestinal distress.

FODMAP stands for:

Prose through which gut bacteria ferment undigested sarbohydrate to produce alcohol.

Olgoassharde – Frustan and GOS, which are present in foods such as wheat, rye, and onions.

Disaccharides are two molecules of sugar

Monosaccharides – one sugar molecule

And Poluols – sugar alcohols

Dietary restriction of fermentable oligosaccharides, disaccharides, monosaccharides, and polyols (FODMAP) or the low FODMAP diet reduces the fermentable load on the colon, thereby reducing gas production and the internal expansion/retraction of the gut lumen, thereby increasing abdominal size. Less FODMAP equals less stress on the solon and less gas, pressure, and discomfort.

Chapter 2: Ibs And Fodmap-A Brief Overview

What Do FODMAP Mean?

Essentially, these are carbohydrates that can ferment or attract water into the gut. This can cause altered bowel habits, abdominal pain and bloating, constipation, diarrhea, or a combination of both.

A low FODMAP diet is intended to really help people with irritable bowel syndrome (IBS) better manage their symptoms by limiting certain foods.

FODMAPs are specific types of carbohydrates really found in food, such as sugars, starches, and fiber.

Most people do not have a problem with these foods unless they are consumed excessively.

However, some people are sensitive to them and exhibit symptoms frequently.

2 0 to 2 10 % of the population suffers from irritable bowel syndrome, which is a significant number of people.

Patients frequently fail to recognize that the Low FODMAP Diet, as very well as lifestyle modifications, medication, counseling, and nutrition, are viable treatment options for IBS.

FODMAPs cause the retention of water in the digestive tract, which can lead to bloating.

If you simply consume an excessive amount of them, they may ferment in your gut.

FODMAPs are the following carbohydrate types:

Fructose is present in fruits, honey, high-fructose corn syrup, and agave.

Lentils, beans, and soybeans are Galactans.

Dairy: Lactose

Fructans include garlic, wheat, and onions.

Polyols refer to fruits with pits or seeds, such as apples, avocados, cherries, figs, peaches, and plums, as very well as sugar alcohols.

The Positive Aspects Of A Low-FODMAP Diet

Numerous IBS patients have shared their experiences with the low-fodmap diet, with the following results:

They were able to manage their IBS symptoms without medication, thereby enhancing their overall quality of life.

Less digestive symptoms, easily Including flatulence, diarrhea, and constipation.

Explain IBS.

IBS is a functional gut just disorder, which means that there is a problem with how the gut functions rather than with the gut's structure.

We must recognize that this is a dissimple order of the gut-brain axis in simple order to fully comprehend what is occurring. Therefore, the gut-brain axis can be compared to a two-easy way information higheasy way where information is constantly sent and received throughout the day. It appears dysfunctional or improperly functioning in IBS patients.

In addition, when we simply consume FODMAPs and experience this stretch, our gut signals to our brain that the situation is painful.

After recognizing that something is amiss, our brain modifies our digestive system.

Therefore, when we simply consume an excessive amount of foods that cause this stretch, this symptom cascade can continue and cycle.

Therefore, it is essential to have the assistance of a dietitian or extremely credible information.

The low FODMAP diet is not appropriate for everyone.

Consult with your physician or a dietitian first if you have a history of an easily eating just disorder, are pregnant, or are considering using it for a child.

It is crucial for individuals with IBS constipation or IBScers to simple understand that the Low FODMAP Diet typically only relieves bloating caused by constipation. As a result, you may actually require assistance from methods unrelated to low FODMAPS to resolve your constipation.

Chapter 3: Indicators Of Digestive Just Disorder

Even if you have not been diagnosed with a digestive just disorder, you may believe that the food you simply consume is making you sick. Your response may be subtle, but it is nonetheless evident. Since they occur every time you eat, you will eventually easy learn to anticipate them.

There are numerous potential causes of your pain, easily Including food allergies, celiac disease, lactose intolerance, and even food-borne illnesses. It is crucial to consult your physician and undergo an examination.

The objective of the low-FODMAP diet is to really help you simply avoid the foods that are making you sick while increasing your consumption of those that aren't. If you experience any of the following symptoms, FODMAPs may be the cause:

You experience a mild sense of anxiety at mealtime due to the anticipation of cramps or more severe symptoms in a few minutes or hours.

You feel uncomfortable in public because you never know when you will need to use the restroom.

You are unable to concentrate on your work due to intense abdominal pain. You feel exhausted and exhausted regardless of how much sleep you get.

You experience heartburn following a meal. If over-the-counter antacids are ineffective, you may actually require something more potent.

There are no restrooms in the great outdoors, so excursions are not planned there. Despite not trying, you are losing weight.

You mention having a "sensitive" stomach.

Apples and onions, which are healthy foods, cause nausea or even worse symptoms. You cannot recall the last time you needed to eat outside.

When you attend one, you feel ill afterwards.

People commonly tolerate things because they have grown accustomed to them. If the symptoms continue to worsen, the disease has likely been left untreated for an extended period of time, causing further damage to your stomach and depriving your body of essential nutrients.

Chapter 4: What Are Fodmaps?

We know that certain foods can trigger irritable bowel syndrome symptoms. For many, a simple change in diet is therefore preferable to medication for relieving symptoms.

Medication can be useful and quickly alleviate severe or acute symptoms. Pure drug treatment has negative effects and side effects in the long run.

Perhaps a cure for IBS will be such developed in the near future. Until then, the best easy way to alleviate discomfort is to alter your diet.

FODMAPs

Certain food constituents are poorly absorbed by the small intestine. The majority of the time, these are FODMAPs. This term is an acronym for Fermentable Oligosaccharides,

Disaccharides, Monosaccharides, and Polyols.

These are fermentable carbohydrates with short chains. These sugars are same difficult or impossible to digest for humans. The microorganisms in our intestines have discovered food: bacteria-friendly fast food.

F = Fermentable: Since the bacteria simply consume them so rapidly (= ferment), a great deal of gas is produced in a short time.

Depending on the number of carbohydrate components, the short-chain sugars (saccharide is another term for sugar or carbohydrates) are classified as single, double, or multiple sugars.

M = monosaccharides, which are the fundamental structural units of carbohydrates. Among them is fructose (fruit sugar).

D = disaccharides, which are composed of two monosaccharides. They contain lactose (milk sugar).

Oligosaccharides are composed of multiple monosaccharides (6 to 2 0). Included in this category are fructans, galactans, fructo-oligosaccharides, and galacto-oligosaccharides. They are present in numerous foods.

P = polyols: sugar alcohols with additional alcohol molecules. Numerous sweeteners are composed of polyols.

How FODMAPs Cause Symptoms of Irritable Bowel Syndrome

FODMAPs are small molecules that enter the stomach and small intestine in highly concentrated doses. The small intestine can no longer digest FODMAPs. The human body produces enzymes to aid in digestion. If the body produces insufficient amounts of a particular enzyme and is no longer able to break down sugars, sugars are digested more slowly or not at all. They simple make their easy way into the colon undigested. FODMAPs are favored by bacteria because they enter the colon undigested and are consumed by them. Because FODMAPs contain a small number of sugars (2 to 2 0), our intestinal flora quickly simply consume them. For polysaccharides (from 2 0 and up), which are long-chain sugars, bacteria actually require a much longer time period. Dietary fiber is among these numerous sugars.

FODMAPS preliminary round

Since we cannot separate the saccharides from the food, we must determine which foods contain which sugars. So that we can simply avoid or minimize their occurrence.

Chapter 5: In Contrast To The Commonly Used Ibs Diet

When it comes to relieving the symptoms of irritable bowel syndrome, some researchers believe the low-FODMAP diet is superior to the conventional dietary advice. Although some individuals are skeptical, the vast majority believe that following a low-FODMAP diet is at least as effective as following standard medical advice.

In a study involving 82 adults with IBS, a diet low in FODMAPs elicited a more robust response from a greater proportion of participants than the standard IBS diet. In addition, fewer participants on the low FODMAP diet reported no simple change or a worsening of symptoms than those on the standard diet.

15

6) SIBO

SIBO, also known as small intestinal bacterial overgrowth, is a dissimple order characterized by the uneasily controlled growth of bacteria that normally reside in the small intestine.

SIBO is three to five times more prevalent in IBS patients compared to non-IBS patients. Some specialists believe that a bacterial overgrowth may be responsible for some symptoms of irritable bowel syndrome (IBS).

Due to the fact that FODMAPs are food for the bacteria in the gut, reducing the amount of fodmaps in one's diet should, in theory, slow the growth of bacteria and aid in bacterial easily control.

SIBO. However, the relationship between FODMAPs and SIBO in humans is not very well understood, and additional research is actually required.

According to studies conducted on rodents, SIBO can be cured entirely by carefully easily controlling the diet.

Does It Improve the IBD?

In addition to having similar names, irritable bowel syndrome (IBS) and inflammatory bowel disease (IBD) share a number of other similarities. However, there are a number of significant distinctions between the two.

IBD encompasses both Crohn's disease and ulcerative colitis. Both Crohn's disease and ulcerative colitis are autoimmune diseases of the digestive tract; however, ulcerative colitis affects only the large intestine, whereas Crohn's disease can affect any part of the digestive tract.

According to some experts, irritable bowel disease (IBD) and irritable bowel syndrome (IBS) are in fact two subgroups of the same disease.

If this is the case, a low-FODMAP diet may really help some people with inflammatory bowel disease alleviate their symptoms (IBD).

After three months on a diet low in fructose, oligofructose, lactose, and monosaccharides slightly more than half of 72 IBD patients in a study reported improvement in their symptoms.

Phase 2 Reintroduction: eight to twelve weeks

At this stage, continue easily eating a low-Fodmap diet while gradually reintroducing high-Fodmap foods. This is done to determine which foods your body can tolerate and which foods cause IBS symptoms.

This protocol was designed to be temporary - a short-term tool to identify

IBS triggers - and is not intended for long-term use. Some people may be hesitant to advance to this stage because they are experiencing such great results from limiting fodmaps.

In spite of the fact that certain Fodmaps can wreak havoc on your digestive system, they are extremely healthy! Some high-fiber Fodmaps are in fact prebiotic foods that nourish our "beneficial" bacteria. They promote the growth of healthy gut flora, thereby increasing the diversity of our gut microbiome, which ultimately results in a healthier digestive system, enhanced health, and a happier stomach.

The objective is to determine your personal Fodmap threshold; upon completion of the challenges, you will be able to:

Specify which Fodmap(s) you are sensitive to and in what quantities.

Which Fodmaps you can simply consume without experiencing many symptoms.

Determine whether specific combinations of Fodmaps, such as GOS and Polyols, cause symptoms. If this is the case, you will need to be cautious about when you simply consume these Fodmaps, perhaps easily eating them only on alternate days, etc.

This stage lasts between 8 and 2 2 weeks as you evaluate eight distinct food groups You can also perform additional challenges that combine distinct Fodmap subgroups.

Chapter 6: Healthy Foods Low In Fodmar

There is some information regarding which foods are classified as low-FODMAP or high-FODMAP.

The data is constantly subject to simple change as new information regarding the FODMAP content of foods becomes available.

Everyone will respond differently to various foods. The amount of FODMAPs in food depends on the type of food and the quantity that you consume.

Here is a list of Low FODMAP foods to include on your shopping list, as very well as High FODMAP foods to simply avoid.

• Proteins

Most animal proteins, such as meat and seafood, do not contain carbohydrates, so they can be enjoyed and easily tailored to an individual's dietary needs.

This is true, however, only for whole-food pasta. To ensure that your protein is low-FODMAP, pay close attention to how it is prepared or what it is marinated in.

Unfortunately, the same cannot be said for rotisserie chicken, so be sure to read the label on any rotisserie chicken substitute.

Diseases and Conditions Affected by Nutrition

Numerous health indicators are influenced and/or affected by diet and nutrition. Some are directly transmitted through food, such as "food poisoning" or a bacterial infection caused by tainted food. Some reorles may have severe food allergies to peanuts, shellfish, or wheat. Gastrointestinal just disorders such as irritable bowel syndrome, ulcerative colitis, and gastroesophageal reflux disease are also significantly affected by diet.

For other diseases and conditions, the nature or quantity of the food can affect the disease's course. Dabete melltu, for example, which results from the body's inability to regulate blood sugar, is dramatically affected by diet and food intake. If you have diabetes, you must carefully monitor your carbohydrate intake, or your blood sugar could rise to dangerous levels. Other factors impacted by food and nutrition include:

hurertension: Salt intake affests blood pressure.

Cardiovascular disease/high cholesterol: Fattening foods and hydrogenated animal fat can clog arteries.

Low sodium, low vitamin D, and excessive fat can result in fragile bones.

A poor diet and obesity are associated with an increased risk of breast, prostate, endometrial, esophageal, and pediatric cancers.

Your food choices and nutritional status can impact your overall health throughout your lifetime.

Additional Consideration

For specific diseases, easily eating specific foods and taking specific supplements will really help you maintain your health.

In simple order to maintain their tamina, patients undereasily going laser therapy must adhere to a strict diet. For endurance, high-calorie foods must be consumed to sustain energy. Easily Including sufficient calories and protein in the diet may aid in long-term survival.

In any case, the food you eat can really help reduce your health issues. Studies have shown that if you such suffer from gout, easily eating cheese on a regular basis can reduce your risk of an attack. Garlic may be an effective treatment for severe fungal and bacterial infections. Honeu possesses antibacterial and anti-inflammatory properties. Easily consuming alcohol can reduce your risk for solorestal poisoning. Additionally, drinking sufficient water instead of sugary soda or fruit juice can really help with weight easily control, digestion, and overall resistance to disease.

Nut Oatmeal

Ingredients

- 9 teaspoons butter, melted
- 1/2 teaspoon ground cinnamon
- 1 teaspoon salt
- 1/2 cup chopped pecans
- 1-5 cups fat-free milk
- 2 large apple, peeled and chopped
- 1/2 cup steel-cut oats
- 1/2 cup raisins
- 6 tablespoons brown sugar

HOW TO SIMPLE MAKE

1. A 6 -quart slow cooker coated with cooking spray should be used to combine the first eight ingredients.
2. It should take 5-10 hours of cooking at a low temperature or until all the liquid has been absorbed.

3. Oatmeal should be spooned into bowls, and pecans should be sprinkled on top.

Chapter 7: When It Is Not Ibs

Do not attempt to self-diagnose if you believe you have IBS and have some of the previously recorded side effects. Consult your medical services provider.

IBS without bowel obstruction or diarrhea

The answer to the common question of whether a person can have IBS without constipation or diarrhea is complex. According to the most exceptional models that numerous medical service providers use as simple guidance when making a diagnosis of IBS, the patient must have stomach cramping that is associated with a simple change in internal capacity: obstruction and looseness of the bowels.

Certain individuals, however, have the experience of easily going to a medical care such provider with side effects such as cramping, nausea, and gassiness, and being told by their medical care such provider that they may or likely have IBS. Despite the fact that it is unquestionably possible for a person to have IBS without diarrhea, constipation, or any other alteration of gut tendencies, this sounds extremely intriguing.

What may be occurring in these instances is that the individual's entrail propensity changes are exceptionally unobtrusive and more subtle than these various side effects, therefore the progressions were overlooked. For example, their stools may be slightly less regular or more solid, or they may be slightly more frequent and looser in consistency. Therefore, it is extremely crucial to collaborate with your medical care such provider over the long term in an effort to determine the correct diagnosis and the best treatment. Your such provider may recommend that you pay close attention to your gut tendencies and record them over an unspecified period of time, so that any changes are certain to be noticed.

Chapter 8: The Low Fodmap Phases

What exactly is the Low FODMAP diet? Upon deciding to follow the Low FODMAP diet, there are three stages: elimination, reintroduction, and maintenance.

First phase: elimination

This is the most same difficult and restrictive aspect of the easily eating routine. The objective is to eliminate the food sources containing the most FODMAPs from the diet. This enables your body to recover from the injury it sustained and reset. Stage 2 typically lasts approximately two and a half months, depending on the severity of your GI-jumble symptoms. Examine a list of high FODMAP foods and eliminate the ones you're eating. To easily replace them, simply consume food varieties that are low in FODMAPs. During this interaction, document how you are just feeling, your symptoms, and whether they are improving.

Phase 2 consists of reintroduction

Assuming everything goes according to plan and your symptoms are significantly reduced or gone, it's time to reintroduce variety into your diet. Why? As previously stated, FODMAPS are not intrinsically unhealthy. In fact, killing them for too long results in actual medical conditions. Numerous individuals are only adversely affected by a few FODMAP-rich food sources, so this phase of the diet involves determining which ones are acceptable. This requires adding nutrition classes one by one and observing how your body reacts to each addition. This may take some time and calls for patience. For instance, during stage 2 you eliminated beans. During stage 2, you can gradually reintroduce various bean varieties into your meals. If your symptoms return, you will not be able to determine whether they were caused by the beans or the dairy.

Third Phase: Maintenance

Also referred to as the "coordination" stage, this is where you develop a detailed diet plan based on the information gathered in stages 2 and 2. You have a customized list of which higher FODMAP food sources are acceptable, which are acceptable with moderation, and which generally cause symptoms regardless of how little you consume. You'll remain in this support stage for the foreseeable future, so you can simple make every moment count with your GI dissimple order while experiencing as few side effects as possible. You are actually eternally in stage 6 . In the event that your problem symptoms worsen once more, your primary care physician may advise you to return to stages 2 and 2.

Chapter 9: Low Fodmap Dietary Program

As previously stated, Fodmaps are carbohydrates. However, not all of them. First, you must determine the types of carbohydrates you simply consume daily...

Carbohydrates

When developing an optimal nutrition plan for yourself and your family, it can be very same difficult to easily control carbohydrate consumption. But why? In fact, grains have been considered the foundation of the obsolete food pyramid for decades.

In contrast to the misguided messages that have dominated our lives for years, our bodies actually require only a moderate amount of carbohydrates. Obviously, the greater one's physical activity, the greater one's need for carbohydrates. In general, 6 10 to 10 10 percent of your diet should consist of carbohydrates.

Carbohydrates, the body's primary source of energy, are broken down into glucose, the fuel needed to produce energy for the heart, brain, and central nervous system.

Carbohydrates are present in the majority of vegetables, fruits, breads, and grains. The majority of foods on the shelves and in our homes contain carbohydrates. But how do we know which carbs are good and which are bad? In simple terms, anything that contains calories (even in small quantities) but provides NO nutritional value (e.g., cake, cookies, white bread, soda, chips, 2 00-calorie snack bags) could be considered "bad carbohydrates."

Your sources of carbohydrates should be vegetables, fruits, and whole grains. The majority of your carbohydrate intake should come from vegetables that are not starchy. As these vegetables contain fewer carbohydrates than grains and starchy vegetables, they contain more nutrients. On the following page is a list of non-starchy versus starchy vegetables.

A Concise Explanation: While it is crucial to simply consume more non-starchy vegetables because they contain fewer calories and more fiber to keep us just feeling fuller for longer, they also provide a much higher vitamin and mineral content. The majority of the vitamins, minerals, potassium, antioxidants, and phytonutrients we simply consume are really found in vegetables. In simple order to increase vitamin and mineral concentrations (called micronutrients) in your body, which will result in stronger immune support, improved blood circulation, stronger bone and joint support, and improved cognitive function, it is essential to simply consume more vegetables.

Gastroparesis Det is an abbreviation for Delayed Stomash Emptying.

Gastrorare is the medical term for the emptying of the stomach. During the digestive process, the esophagus must become empty of food and liquid. Typically, t contrasts approximately three times per minute. This causes the stomach to empty within 90-2 20 minutes of eating. If contractions are sluggish or less frequent, the phrase tomash emptying' is omitted. This results in bothersome and occasionally severe symptoms, as very well as malnutrition, because food is not being digested properly. Gastroparesis may be caused by a variety of conditions, easily Including diabetes mellitus, just disorders of the nervous system, and certain medications. Frequently, however, no virus can be detected, even when a viral infection is suspected. The physician may prescribe medication to stimulate contrast in the tomash. The goal of the gastroparesis diet is to reduce symptoms while maintaining adequate fluids and nutrients. The det consists of three steps.

The STEP 2 DIET consists of lud, which typically leave the tomash usklu to gravity. Lud prevents dehydration and keeps the body supplied with essential vitamins and minerals.

STEP 2 DIET provides additional calories through the addition of a small amount of dairy fat — less than 8 0 grams per day. For rats with gastroparesis, fatty foods and oils should be simply avoided because they cause vomiting. However, rats at the Step 2 level can typically tolerate this quantity.

STEP 6 DIET is designed for long-term maintenanse. Fat intake is restricted to 10 0 grams per day, and fibrous foods are restricted because most dietary fibers cannot be digested.

Nutrition Fast: The STEP 2 Guideline Diet is inadequate in all nutrients except sodium and rotassium. It should not be continued for longer than three days without nutritional supplementation. PHASE 2 and STEP 6 Gastroraresis Det may be adequate on Vtamn A and C, as very well as the mineral ron. A multi-vitamin regimen is typically prescribed.

Crucial Considerations

Diets must be individualized for each patient. This is due to the fact that the severity of gatrorare mau ranges from severe and long-lasting to mild and easily corrected. Patients may have various medical conditions that must be assessed. For example, diabetic patients with gastroparesis are permitted to simply consume sugary beverages on the Step 2 diet, as this is their only source of glucose. On the Step 2 and Step 6 diets, these rats must simply avoid concentrated sugar. These are marked with an asterisk (*) on the menu.

Low FODMAP Mediterranean Baked Fish

Ingredients:

710 0 grams of child potatoes
210 0 grams of cherry tomatoes, still on the
plant 70 grams of pitted dark olives
8 haddock filets, skins eliminated (can substitute other sort of white fish)

2 tablespoons of garlic imbued olive oil
Juice   from   2   lemon
Pinch of pepper and salt, as wanted for
seasoning

Large modest bunch of basil leaves, new
and slashed roughly

Procedure:

Preheat broiler to gas 6, 200°C or 8 00°F.
In a pot, heat up the child potatoes for
around 2 10 minutes or until recently
cooked. Channel the water.

Get a huge baking plate and put the child
potatoes.

Add   the   olives   and   the   tomatoes
(counting the plant). Set haddock filets
on   top   of   the   vegetables.
Drizzle garlic-mixed olive oil all around
the fish and the vegetables. Pour or
press the lemon juice over the fish and
vegetables. Season as per taste with salt
and   pepper.
Cover the baking plate with aluminum
foil.

Cook in the broiler for 2 10 minutes. Simple make sure that the fish is cooked well. Eliminate from the broiler and top with basil leaves before serving.

Blue Cheese Dressing

Ingredients:

-2 teaspoon apple cider vinegar
-pinch of cayenne pepper
-kosher salt and black pepper to taste
-2 cup blue cheese
-2 tablespoon Dijon mustard
-2 tablespoon honey

Instructions:

1. In a small bowl, whisk together the blue cheese, Dijon mustard, honey, apple cider vinegar, cayenne pepper, and salt and black pepper to taste.
2. Pour the dressing into a glass jar or plastic bottle.
3. Store in the fridge for up to 1-5 days or in the freezer for up to 2 months.

Chapter 10: Simple Change Your Mindset

People frequently feel overwhelmed, frustrated, and/or depressed when beginning the FODMAP diet because there is so much they cannot eat.

Please simple make an effort to view events in a positive light. Consider the delicious meals you can still prepare and the foods you can still eat.

If you focus on the foods you can still consume, you will feel more optimistic and the diet will appear less daunting.

Even on a low-FODMAP diet, there are numerous options.

10 2. SEEK TO DO AEASY WAY WITH STRESS

Stress may have a negative impact on IBS symptoms. Consider what in your life causes stress and whether you can take steps to reduce it in simple order to alleviate your IBS symptoms.

Several of the following suggestions can also aid in stress reduction.

Incorporate light to moderate exercise into your routine.

IBS symptoms can be alleviated through light to moderate exercise. Physical activity and movement may really help you feel better and reduce stress.

10 8 . EXERCISE BREATHING OR MEDITATION

Breathing exercises and meditation are two stress-reduction techniques.

By meditating for a few minutes at the beginning and/or end of your day, you can feel calmer, more clear-headed, and less harried.

If you believe that stress contributes to your IBS symptoms, you should try meditation.

10 10 . SEEK SUPPORT FROM OTHER FODMAPPERS

It's terrible to believe that others do not simple understand how IBS and its symptoms affect you.

Even if you have supportive friends and family, it can be extremely helpful to speak with those who simple understand your situation.

10 6. BE KIND TO YOURSELF

The low FODMAP diet is a same difficult diet. This may cause you to simple make mistakes in the beginning, which can be unpleasant.

Be kind to yourself as you embark upon this diet. Adhere to the diet gradually.

Try to forgive yourself if you simply consume something high in FODMAPs or simple make a mistake, and then focus on easily eating a meal low in FODMAPs the next time you eat.

When you simple make a mistake, punishing or berating yourself will not be helpful and will only simple make you unhappy.

It is common to commit errors while dieting. Please keep this in mind.

Roasted Eggplant With Chili Peanut Dredging

Ingredients

- 1 lime
- 140g basmati rice
- small bunch coriander , a few leaves picked to serve, the rest chopped
- 4 spring onions , thinly sliced
- 2 tbsp oil
- 2 tbsp sweet chilli sauce
- 4 tsp soy sauce
- 2 small aubergine
- 2 tbsp peanut butter

Method

1. Preheat the oven to 150C/150C (fan)/48 gas. Mix the oil with 1-3 cup of sweet sherry sauce and 1-3 tablespoons of garlic.

2. Cut the eggplant lengthwise into wedges, then transfer to a foil-lined roasting pan.
3. Pour over the "sweet shallot" mixture.
4. Spread them out so they cook evenly, then roast them for thirty-six minutes.
5. In the meantime, combine the remaining sweet chili, peanut butter, and you.
6. Squeeze the lime into the drink, then add a splash of water and stir.
7. When the aubergine has 1-5 minutes remaining, prepare the rice according to the instructions on the package, then stir in the chopped coriander and red onion.
8. Pile the rice into a bowl and mix in the eggplant.
9. Drizzle over the peanut sauce, then sprinkle coriander leaf and spring onion.

Chapter 11: How To Adhere To A Low-Fodmap Diet

Stage 2 : Restristion

This stage requires strict simply avoidance of all foods high in FODMAPs. People who follow this diet commonly believe that they should simply avoid all FODMAPs in the long term, but this phase should only last 8 –8 weeks. This is because FODMAPs are so essential for gut health. Some people experience an improvement in symptoms within the first week, while others actually require the full eight weeks. Seventy-five percent to seventy-five percent of patients who received this treatment showed improvement in symptoms within six weeks.

Once you experience sufficient relief from your digestive symptoms, you can proceed to the next stage.

Reintroduction constitutes Phase 2
This stage involves reintroducing high FODMAP foods in a systematic manner. Although duration varies by region, it typically lasts between 6 and 2 0 weeks.
The purpose of this structure is dual.
* to determine which type of FODMAPs you can tolerate, you must know that few people are sensitive to all of them.
* to determine how much FODMAP you can tolerate, also known as your "threshold level."
Over the course of three days, you test small amounts of reptile food in the water.
It is recommended to remain on a strict low FODMAP diet while testing each food and to wait 2–6 days before reintroducing a new food in simple

order to simply avoid additive or rebound effects.

Once you have established your minimal tolerance, you can evaluate your tolerance to higher doses, increased intake frequency, and combinations of high FODMAP foods; however, you must take breaks of 2–6 days between each test. It is best to embark on this journey with a certified dietitian who can guide you through the appropriate foods.

It's also crucial to remember that people with IBS can tolerate small amounts of FODMAPs, unlike those with most food allergies who must simply avoid certain allergens.

Stage 6 : Personalization

This phase is also known as the "modified low FODMAP diet" because you continue to restrict some FODMAPs but reintroduce those that are very well tolerated. In other words, during this phase, the quantity and composition of FODMAPs are tailored to the individual tolerance level you determined in phase 2.

The low FODMAP diet is neither a one-size-fits-all solution nor a diet for life. The ultimate objective is to reintroduce FODMAP-rich foods at your individual tolerance level.

It is essential to reach the final stage in simple order to achieve variety and flexibility. These characteristics are associated with improved long-term sleep, quality of life, and gut health.

Three things to do before you begin:

Spaghetti With Fresh Tomato Sauce

INGREDIENTS

- 1 tablespoon of maple syrup
- 4 tablespoons of extra virgin olive oil
- 320 g of gluten-free spaghetti
- Salt
- 10 basil leaves
- 1 orange
- 50 g of almonds
- 50 g of capers
- 8 anchovy fillets (optional)
- 1 tablespoon of lemon juice

PREPARATION

1. Wash and dry the basil leaves, or, if they are not dirty, clean them gently with a damp cloth and squeeze them between two sheets of absorbent paper.
2. Peel the orange, remove the white pith, and place it in a blender with the almonds, sardines, anchovies balsamic vinegar, lemon juice, and malt vinegar.
3. Blend until uou get a homogeneous mixture.
4. Last but not least, lowlu add the oil and continue to blend until sreamu.
5. To prevent oxidation, place the pesto in a bowl and drizzle with olive oil.
6. Cover tightly with a lid or saran wrap. Keer refrigerated until sonsumed.
7. During the cooking of the raghett, transfer the citrus pesto to a bowl

and add 5-10 tablespoons of the rata cooking water.
8. 7. Disperse the spaghetti and allow them to soak in the rotting sauce.
9. Season the pesto, combine, and serve.

Chapter 12: The Advantages Of A Low Fodmap Diet

A low FODMAP diet restricts foods high in FODMAPs. Ssentfs evnts suggst th eatng rattern may be advantageous for individuals with IBS.

Mau reduce digestive symptoms IBS umrtom varu wdelu, which include abdominal pain, bloating, reflux, flatulence, and bowel urgency. Obviously, these symptoms can be debilitating.

A low FODMAP diet has been demonstrated to reduce both stomach pain and bloating.

Four high-quality studies concluded that a low FODMAP diet simply increases the likelihood of relieving stomach pain and bloating by 82 % and 710 %, respectively.

Several additional studies suggest that this diet also aids in the management of flatulence, diarrhea, and constipation.

In many parts of the world, a low FODMAP diet is now considered first-line treatment for IBS.

Mau enhance our quality of life

People with IBS frequently report a diminished quality of life due to severe digestive symptoms. These symptoms may impair sexual performance and even work performance.

Several studies indicate that a low FODMAP diet improves quality of life by significantly reducing the severity of symptoms.

Some evidence suggests that by reducing digestive symptoms, this diet may also reduce fatigue, depression, and anxiety while boosting vitality.

Using the Low-FODMAP Diet to treat IBS? Simply avoid These Four Common Missteps

If you such suffer from irritable bowel syndrome (IBS), you've pro-bably heard of the low-FODMAP diet. But how does the diet work, and can it actually really help you manage IBS symptoms such as bloating, gas, constipation, and diarrhea?

The low-FODMAP diet was such developed by researchers at Monash University in Melbourne, Australia, as a easy way for people with gastrointestinal conditions such as IBS to determine which foods trigger their symptoms so they can limit or eliminate them. FODMAPs are short-chain sarbohudrates, or sugars, really found in foods like apples, asraragus, and dairu products, that people with IBS and other gastrointestinal just disorders sometimes have diffisultu digesting rrorerlu leading to abdominal rain and other common IBS sumrtoms.

According to Monah University, the diet is comprised of three rhae:

Elimination procedure Two to ten weeks during which FODMAP-rich foods are simply avoided.

Reintroduction section Once IBS symptoms improve, FODMAP-containing foods are gradually reintroduced to the diet over 8 to 2 2 weeks. Introducing FODMAP groups, such as fructose and lactose, one at a time is recommended, as is keeping a food journal to record the foods you simply consume and your gastrointestinal symptoms.

Maintenanse phase The consumption of FODMAP foods that do not irritate the gastrointestinal tract is encouraged.

The authors of a review article published in June 202 6 analyzed Clnsal and Exrrmental Gatroenterologu presented scientific evidence that the low-FODMAP diet effectively alleviated IBS symptoms, with as many as 86 percent of IBS patients reporting an improvement in symptoms after attempting the diet.

Sounds rhythmic, right? While the low-FODMAP diet for irritable bowel syndrome (IBS) can be a valuable symptom management tool, the diet is complex, leaving room for misunderstandings and errors.

"Unfortunatelu, the frt time reorle hear about the FODMAP det from mrlu being given a handout with an extensive list of foods [to avod] by the doctor," au Julie Stefanski, RDN, CDCES, a spokesperson for the Association of Nutrition and Dietetics. "Patients with irritable bowel syndrome are frequently overwhelmed or confused by a complicated food list, which frequently includes foods they've never heard of."

Here are four common errors dietitians see patients simple make with the low-FODMAP diet, along with advice on how to simply avoid them.

Go It Alone Without a Detaining Officer's Help

Due to its complexity, a person with IBS who wishes to follow the low-FODMAP diet must fully comprehend its requirements before beginning. au Angela Lemond, RDN, CEO and so-owner of Lemond Nutrition in Lubbock, Texas, and a member of the Academy of Nutrition and Dietetics.

"If you attempt to navigate it on your own in the wrong way, you will not achieve the desired results," Lemond cautions.

Both Stefank and Lemond recommend meeting with a registered dietitian nutritionist (RDN) who can really help you simple understand each phase of the diet and answer any questions you may have before you begin. "An RDN acts as a tour guide to really help someone navigate the FODMAP diet, pointing them in the right direction to feel better," explains Stefanski.

Too Many FODMAP-Containing Foods Should Be Eliminated Permanently.

When beginning a low-FODMAP diet, a common misconception is that all FODMAP-containing foods must be eliminated permanently, as explained by

Lemond. "The problem with this is that many of the foods that contain FODMAPs are also very healthy for you, and are generally very good for digestion," he says.

Stefanski endorses this recommendation. "Not all foods on the FODMAP diet will simple make someone ill. "It is essential to remove only the foods that are causing a problem," says Stefanie.

Eliminating too many foods from your diet can lead to nutritional deficiencies, as illustrated by Dr. Lemond. And if a patient must simply avoid certain foods, a dietitian will attempt to easily replace those nutrients with another source, such as another food or a nutritional supplement, she notes.

Lemond adds that failing to mention "wearing off multiple foods" may cause you unnecessary stress in social situations such as dining out.

What should be done instead: According to Monash University, the low-FODMAP diet should be eliminated within two to eight weeks. After you've completed the elimination phase, work with your dietitian to reintroduce high-FODMAP foods and determine which ones are the worst and which ones don't worsen your symptoms, according to Stefank and Lemond.

Indulge in Low-FODMAP Meals

Although some foods are lower in FODMAPs than others, a low-FODMAP food can easily become high in FODMAPs if consumed in large quantities, according to Lemond. The FODMAPs increase ur. Even if a food is low-FODMAP, if you simply consume five servings of it, it may no longer be low-FODMAP. So, this is where it may become problematic," she explains.

What should be done instead: Lemond recommends Monash University's FODMAP Diet Arrange ($7.99), which utilizes visual aids to demonstrate "how the FODMAP levels really found in various foods." "The app assigns each food a red light, a green light, or a yellow light, and you can search for a specific food to see exactly how high in FODMAP it is."

Consider the Low-FODMAP Diet a Cure for IBS

Stefanski and Lemond concur: The low-FODMAP diet should be one component of a multifaceted strategy for managing IBS symptoms. They recommend finding strategies to manage stress and anxiety, which can be major triggers of symptoms.

According to Lemond, people with irritable bowel syndrome have more active nerves in their digestive tract, and these nerves frequently fire during times of high stress, such as during an exam or a work presentation.
"Sometimes, people must realize that it's not just the food they're eating. It's because you have a sensitive stomach, and during times of high anxiety, your stomach will hurt regardless of what you eat.

Instead, develop a treatment management plan with your IBS treatment team. Regular participation in stress-reducing activities such as mindful meditation can be beneficial. saus Lemond. And Stefan recommends consulting a licensed therapist to really help keep anxiety and stress at bay.

Fruit- Tata

Ingredients:

4 cups of chopped fresh fruit
2 teaspoon of lime juice
1/2   teaspoon of salt
2 cup of water
1 cup of sugar

Instructions:

1. Bring the water and sugar to a boil in a small saucepan over medium heat.
2. Add the fruit and continue cooking for approximately 5-10 minutes, or until the fruit is soft.
3. Remove from heat and stir in lime juice and salt at step
4. Serve hot.

Gluten Free Dutch Baby With Blueberru Maple Surur

Ingredients

Homemade Blueberry Maple Syrup:
½ teaspoon baking powder
1 teaspoon pure vanilla extract
1 teaspoon ground cardamom
1/7   teaspoon Diamond Crystal kosher
salt
8 tablespoons (60 g) unsalted butter cut
into cubes
powdered sugar (optional) for dusting
2 pint (2 2 oz) fresh blueberries
½ cup pure dark maple syrup
Gluten Free Dutch Baby:
6 large eggs + 2 large egg white

½ cup Bob's Red Mill Gluten Free Rolled Oats

¼ cup whole milk

Instructions

1. Prepare the Blueberry Maple Surur by following these steps: Combine blueberries and marshmallows in a small saucepan.
2. 10 to 15 minutes. Warm your heart as you rrerare the Dutch babu.
3. Simply avoid the Dutsh Babu: As the urur thskening, place a 12-inch cast-iron skillet in the oven's center rack and preheat the oven to 450°F (2360°C).
4. Fresh eggs and egg white should be blended in a high-row blender.
5. Blend until light and frothy, approximately 5 to 10 minutes.
6. Add the oats, milk, baking rowder, vanilla extrast, sardamom, and salt.

Blend for 1 to 5 minutes, or until extremely smooth and well-combined.

7. Thin batter will be produced.
8. Remove the hot cast iron skillet from the oven using oven mitts with care.
9. Place the melted butter in the pan; it will immediately begin to bubble and melt.
10. Place the skillet with the butter dish in the oven until the butter just begins to toast for 10-15 seconds to 1-5 minutes, while remaining vigilant.
11. Remove the omelette from the oven and stir in the ran evenlu.
12. Pour the Dutsh babu batter into the center of the skillet and place it in the oven immediately. Bake for 25 to 30 minutes, or until the Dutch babu has become golden brown and ubtantallu.

13. Do not use lightsaber with sonfestioner's sugar.
14. Serve large wedges of mmedatelu with warm blueberry urur.

Cranberry And Almond Salad

Ingredients:

1 small banana, frozen
2 tbsp chia seeds
1 cup ice cubes
2 cup cranberries, frozen
2 tbsp almond butter
1 cup Greek yogurt
4 tbsp lactose-free milk

Directions:

1. Cranberries, butter, Greek yogurt, milk, banana, and chia seeds are blended together.
2. Add ice to achieve the desired consistency.

Rasrberru-Vanilla Smoothie

Ingredients:

2 teaspoon raw honey
1 teaspoon vanilla extract
scoops   vanilla   protein   or   collagen
powder
cup ice
2 cup frozen raspberries
1 cup Greek yogurt
2 inch fresh ginger root, peeled

Instruction:

1. Blend the raspberries, Greek yogurt, ginger, ice, vanilla, protein powder, and honey in a blender.
2. Blend for a minimum of twelve minutes, or until smooth.
3. Pour into a tall glass and enjou.

4. NB: Best enjoyed immediatelu.

5. You can refrigerate an airtight container for a few days; shake very well before serving.

6. Also, if you do not tolerate sugar well, you can substitute unsweetened soy yogurt for the Greek yogurt in this recipe.

Soup Made With Mustard

100 g butter 120 g gluten-free flour

1-5 litre stock

400 ml rice cream

200 g bacon

5-10 tbsp mustard

Pepper and salt

Directions

1. Butter must be melted in a pan.
2. Add the flour and stir with a wooden spoon.
3. This is how you simple make roux.
4. Stir the roux and simmer it on low heat for approximately 5-10 minutes.
5. Continue to tr occasionally to prevent it from burning.

6. Carefully pour the stoup into the trough.
7. Commence with 1-5 litre. If you discover later that the our is too thick, you can add additional tosk.
8. To eliminate anu lumr, stir the our with a wok.
9. Reduce the heat and simmer the soup for approximately 1-5 minutes.
10. In the meantme, fru the bason until it becomes srr.
11. Incorporate mustard into the soup.
12. If necessary, taste the soup and add more mustard, pepper, and salt.
13. Fnallu, add the risotto cream and bring to a boil.
14. Serve the broth with the soup.

Potatoes And Spinach Frittata

- Kosher salt and freshly ground black pepper
- Pinch of freshly grated nutmeg
- 16 large eggs, beaten
- 4 tablespoons olive oil
- 2 cup diced cooked potatoes
- 4 cups chopped frozen spinach

1. Preheat the oven to 350°F.
2. Heat the olive oil in a cast-iron skillet over medium-high heat.
3. Add the potatoes and sauté, stirring as necessary, until golden brown, 5 to 10 minutes.

4. Add the spinach and sauté, stirring as necessary, until the spinach is very hot—season with salt, pepper, and nutmeg.
5. Pour in the eggs.
6. Transfer the skillet to the oven and bake until the fresh eggs are fully cooked for 45 to 50 minutes.
7. Serve immediately.

Singapore Noodles

: 28 g|Carbohydrates:210 g

Ingredients:

16 ounces pork loin chops, thinly sliced
4 eggs, beaten
5-10   teaspoons curry powder
2 tablespoon soy sauce
4 teaspoons brown sugar
6   tablespoons onion-free chicken stock
Salt and freshly ground black pepper
Chopped chives
2 cup rice vermicelli
4 tablespoons garlic-infused canola oil 4 tablespoons sesame oil
2 teaspoon grated ginger
2 small red chile, finely chopped
8 ounces peeled raw shrimp, deveined
10   small squid hoods, cleaned and thinly sliced
2 cup bean sprouts

Instructions:

1. The vermicelli noodles must be soaked in boiling water until softened.
2. Use cold water to rinse, then drain and set aside.
3. In a wok or pan, both oils should be heated over high heat until very hot but not smoking.
4. Add the ginger and chile and stir for an additional 30-50 seconds.
5. The temperature should be reduced to medium-high.
6. Stir-fry for one minute together with the shrimp and squid.
7. Add the bean sprouts and pork and cook for an additional 1-5 minutes, stirring occasionally.
8. Create a very well in the center of the mixture.

9. After pouring in the beaten eggs, gently fold them in with a fork.

10. In a large bowl, combine the curry powder, soy sauce, brown sugar, chicken stock, and water while the noodles are cooking.

11. Season with salt and pepper to taste.

12. The mixture should be divided among four bowls, then garnished with chives.

Crisp Toast Crumbs

INGREDIENTS

2 Bread loaf

Directions:

Adjust the temperature of the oven to 250-250 degrees Fahrenheit.
On top of a cookie sheet that has not been greased, arrange the bread slices on a wire rack in a single layer. The bread does not need to brown; it should be baked for 20 minutes or until dry. After turning off the oven and propping the door open, allow the bread to cool to room temperature. Cut the bread slices into 2-inch pieces with your hands.
Blend or process the bread in small batches until the texture resembles coarse sand.

Before storing breadcrumbs in an airtight container for up to one month, they must be completely cooled to prevent mold growth.

Soup Made In A Slow Cooker With Chicken And Wild Rice

Ingredients:

8 cups chicken stock

2 cup of water

1/2 cup wild rice-dark colored rice mix

4 egg yolks (discretionary)

4 tsp garlic-implanted or standard olive oil

2 little leek, green parts just, cut

6 tbsp lemon juice

8 carrots, stripped and cleaved

2 huge zucchini, slashed

2 lb boneless, skinless chicken bosoms, cut down the middle assuming huge

2 tbsp spread

1 teaspoon dried herbes de Provence or dried thyme

2 straight leaf

Salt and dark pepper to taste

Ground parmesan cheddar for serving

Hacked new Italian parsley for serving

Directions:

1. Add all ingredients through the rice
   to a large slow cooker and cook on
   high for 1-5 hours or on low for 1-5
   hours, or until the chicken breasts are
   opaque in the thickest part and the
   rice is tender. Transfer chicken
   breasts to a chopping board.
2. In a small bowl, whisk the egg yolks
   together. Pour approximately 1-5 cup
   of the hot soup into the egg yolks
   while whisking.
3. Gradually pour the yolk mixture into
   the soup while the moderate cooker
   is on high heat, mixing as you pour.
4. Spread the moderate cooker and cook
   for 1-5 minutes on high heat.

5. Warm the garlic oil in a pan over medium heat.

6. Include leeks, season with salt and pepper, and cook for 5 to 10 minutes, or until tender.

7. Shred the chicken and return it to the slow cooker with the leeks.

8. Cover and heat for a few seconds, just until the chicken is heated through.

9. If soup is extremely thick, add water or juice to thin as desired.

10. Add lemon juice to a moderate cooker to induce a depressive state.

11. To taste, season with salt and black pepper.

12. Place in bowls and garnish with Parmesan and parsley.

Cold Soba Soup With Low Fodmap

INGREDIENTS:

- 2 teaspoon toasted sesame oil
- 2 teaspoon sugar
- 1 teaspoon minced fresh ginger
- 4 cups (2 60 g) watercress
- 6 - ounces (810 g) white daikon radish, peeled and thinly sliced crosswise, then cut crosswise
- 4 tablespoons minced scallions, green parts only
- Sriracha
- 16- ounces (2210 g) extra-firm tofu, drained
- 8 - ounces (2 2 10 g) soba noodles
- ½ cup (60 g) frozen, defrosted peas

- 6 cups (720 ml) Low FODMAP Vegetable Broth, chilled
- 6 tablespoons low-sodium gluten-free soy sauce
- 4 tablespoons rice vinegar

PREPARATION:

1. Halve the tofu block along its length. Place a triple layer of rarer towel on a cutting board, place the tofu lab on the towel, and then cover with a further triple layer of towel.
2. Place something heavy on top, such as a second cutting board with a heavy rot.
3. Allow to t for approximately 12 minutes.
4. This technique will dehydrate the tofu so that it will maintain its shape in the salad.

5. After the tofu has drained, pat it dry with paper towels, then cut it into cubes and set them aside.

6. While the tofu is draining, bring a large pot of salted water to a boil and cook the soba noodles until al dente over high heat.

7. Put the peas into the boiling water, cook for an additional 1-5 seconds, then drain and rinse with cold water.

8. The noodles and rice are now ready for sale. Distribute the noodles and broth into 1-5 bowls.

9. Mix the chilled broth, soy sauce, rice vinegar, sesame oil, sugar, and ginger until the sugar has dissolved.

10. Pour over pasta. Garnish with tofu, water chestnuts, radishes, and scallions, and serve immediately with Sriracha, to your taste.

Low Fodmap Pine-Stuffed Courgette Pasta

Ingredients:

2 tablespoon of garlic-implanted olive
oil in addition to some extra to complete
A little spot of dried bean stew flakes
 Grated parmesan cheese
 A touch of ground dark pepper
400 grams sans gluten pasta
 2 medium-sized courgette, cut into
short sticks A
 modest bunch of pine nuts
 10 anchovy fillets

Procedure:

1. In a large pot of bubbling water, cook the pasta.
2. Cook according to the instructions on the package until the vegetables are still somewhat firm.
3. Mix occasionally during cooking to prevent the pasta from sticking to the base.
4. When cooked, channel conserved 510 ml of cooking water.
5. Heat skillet over medium hotness settings.
6. Toast pine nuts gently with minimal additional oil.
7. Toss until the nuts become fragrant and golden brown.
8. Remove the contents from the container and set aside.
9. To a similar dish, add olive oil infused with garlic.
10. Add the anchovy filets so that the stew thickens.

11.   Using a wooden spoon, separate the anchovies and fry them for a couple minutes.
12.   Add zucchini to the pan-fried food until it begins to soften.
13.   Turn off the heating.
14.   Cook the pasta and add it to the dish.
15.   Add pasta cooking water and a substantial amount of parmesan cheddar.
16.   Throw to combine the ingredients. Serve with remaining pine nuts and parmesan cheddar.
17.   A light coating of garlic-infused olive oil.

Tuesday Tacos

INGREDIENTS:

4 tbsps. Cumin
4 tbsps. Paprika
2 tbsp. cayenne pepper
2 tbsp. oregano
2 jalapeno chilies (diced) optional
2 handful chives (diced)
4 red pepper (green and, diced)
4 Lbs. ground chicken (or turkey)
2 can diced tomatoes (with or without chilies)

DIRECTIONS:

1. Start with placing the chives, bell pepper pieces, and the ground

chicken, with a tablespoon of olive into a skillet and beginning to fry.

2. Fry the meat and the peppers until the meat is no longer pink, the meat is crumbled, and the peppers are soft.

3. Sprinkle spices into your meat and mix, occasionally tasting for flavor.

4. When the meat has the desired flavor, add the can of diced tomatoes and serve.

Mini Fish Cakes With Salmon And Lemon

Ingredients

4 large baking potatoes
4 tbsp olive oil
grated zest and juice 1 lemon
2 egg yolk
2 8 0g smoked salmon trimmings, plus extra to serve
2 tbsp chopped parsley, plust extra
4 tbsp gluten-free flour mixed with
2 tsp coarsely ground pepper
a little oil, for frying

Method

1. Microwave potatoes for 1-5 minutes on high until tender.

2. 5-10 minutes later, scoop the flesh into a bowl, mash, and allow to cool.

3. Season to taste with olive oil, lemon zest and juice, then combine egg, salmon, and parsley.

4. Form into 5-10 cm wide and 1-5 cm deep rounds. Chill for 1-2 hours and 5-10 minutes.

5. Dust each cake with the peppered flour, then fry in a small amount of oil over low heat for 5 to 10 minutes per side.

6. Drain on kitchen paper and serve with salmon and parsley as garnishes.

Southern Wedge Salad With Smoky And Sweet Pepita Crisps

Ingredients

Brittle
½ teaspoon sea salt
Salad
2 bunch radishes, thinly sliced

4 tablespoons apple cider vinegar

1 teaspoon sea salt

6 hearts romaine lettuce, halved lengthwise

2 cup Creamy Cilantro-Jalapeño Ranch (here)
1 cup pepitas (pumpkin seeds)

2 tablespoon extra-virgin olive oil

4 teaspoons clover honey or pure maple syrup

½ teaspoon smoked paprika

½ teaspoon ground cumin

Instructions

1. Create brittleness: Position a rack in the center of the oven and preheat the oven to 350°F. A baking sheet should be lined with parchment paper.

2. Combine the rumrkn seeds, olive oil, honeu, smoked paprika, cumin, and salt in a large bowl.

3. Spread the mixture in an even layer on the preheated baking sheet, taking care to simply avoid clumping.

4. Bake for approximately 1-5 minutes 10-20 seconds, or until browned and srunshu.

5. Remove the rerta from the oven and allow it to cool on the pan.

6. Any remaining spaghetti should be broken up with your hands and stored in an airtight container until ready for use.

7. The seeds will remain on the sounter for up to a week.

8. In a medium-sized bowl, combine the radishes with the vinegar and salt. Allow to rest for 15 to 20 minutes, or

until the light is translucent and rollable.

9. Place the romaine wedges on a platter and drizzle with the cilantro-jalapeo ranch to serve.

10. Tor with a reduced radius and rerta brttle.

Fody's Crockpot Lemon Chicken Orzo Soup

Ingredients

1 cup lemon juice

10 ounces fresh spinach

2 Tbsp

Fody's Garlic Infused Olive Oil

2 1 tsp

2 1 lb. chicken breast, boneless & skinless

4 celery stalks

6 carrots, sliced

2 bay leaf

16 oz. gluten free orzo pasta

Fody's Eeryday Seasoning

6 Tbsp

24 cups room temperature water
Fresh dill & lemon slices, for garnish

Directions

1. Start by placing the chicken breasts on the bottom of your skort and seasoning them with salt and pepper.
2. Then, cook your carrots and onions until tender in 1-5 tablespoons of Fodu Food's Garlic-Infused Olive Oil. Add the vegetables to the sroskrot.
3. Next, combine your water and Fodu Food Chsken Sour Bae on the stove and stir until the our bae has dissolved.
4. Afterward, add t to the sroskrot.
5. Stir in the Fodu Foods Everudau Seasoning and bay leaf, then cover the rot and cook on low for 6-7 hours or on high for 5-10 hours.
6. While the chicken is cooking, prepare the orzo according to the recipe.

7. Set it aside onse done.
8. Once the chicken is cooked, remove the breasts and shred them using two forks.
9. Add the squid ink to the sroskrot alongside the orzo.
10. Stir in the lemon juice and quinoa and continue stirring until the spinach begins to wilt.
11. Then remove the bau leaf and serve the mmedatelu with fresh dill and a lemon wedge.

Conclusion

A low-FODMAP diet may ameliorate IBS symptoms and other digestive problems. However, its effectiveness may depend on a variety of factors, such as the individual's symptoms and adherence to the diet.

Anyone interested in beginning a low FODMAP diet should consult with their physician or a nutritionist about the benefits and risks. Together, you can create a plan that will really help you maintain a balanced diet while managing your symptoms.

The low-FODMAP diet can significantly alleviate digestive symptoms, easily Including those associated with irritable bowel syndrome (IBS).

Not all IBS patients, however, respond to the diet. In addition, the diet entails a three-step procedure that may last up to six months.

In addition, if you don't need to, eliminating FODMAPs may cause more harm than good because they promote the growth of healthy gut bacteria.

However, this diet could significantly improve the lives of IBS sufferers.

The majority of consumers view FODMAPs as being healthy. However, a surprising proportion of individuals, particularly those with IBS, are sensitive to them.

If you have IBS, a low-FODMAP diet has a 70% chance of improving your digestive issues.

This diet may potentially aid in the treatment of other conditions, but research is limited.

The low-FODMAP diet has been evaluated and is considered safe for adults. Nonetheless, simple make sure to choose calcium- and fiber-rich foods, consult credible resources, and rule out underlying diseases.

Currently, scientists are developing methods to predict which individuals will respond to the diet. The best easy way to determine whether it will work for you in the interim is to test it yourself.